PLANT BASED DIET

Lectin Free Recipies Book To Lose Weight And Feel Good

By Holly R. Evans

Contents

Chapter 1:
Introduction

Introduction

As we all know that health is the most important for every living being. It is not merely important for human beings but it is also important for animals and other living creatures of the earth. No matter where a creature or living being exists or live on the earth but health means a lot to everyone. Healthy, physically and mentally fit person is far better than mentally and physically disturbed man, poor health may also cause damage to the brain, thinking capacity and also can become the reason of damage to other body parts.

Mostly we are not used to watch news channels and are also not interested to listen to the news because most of the time there are fake news, which have no strong base and are not based on facts and figures. And most of the time, we are aware of the fact that this news which are being podcasting is not based on truth and has no factual base. So, most of the time we used to avoid to listen such news which are not based on facts and figures.

Degrees also does not matter if you have no knowledge regarding your subject and also in other regards such as health, fitness, selection of healthy food, and also in other aspects of life. One should be aware of the fact that what a healthy diet and health is. Health matters a lot to everyone in one's life. So, one should be able to choose his diet plan or chart. One should be aware of the fact that what a healthy diet is and how much does it matter. Health means a lot to everyone but some are aware of this fact and some are not aware of this fact that health matters a lot. They will care about health when they lose it. Once they lose health than they all came to know that what health actually is and how much does it matter to living beings especially to human life.

Lectin proves life threatening. It causes seriously illness and also become the cause of death for majority. The use of lectin causes serious damage to health and it is also much harmful to human health and human life.

Most of the health experts are of the view that the main cause of illness and laziness is the consumption and intake of fast food and all other nutrition less food. This is the main cause of laziness and also cause serious threat to life. It causes serious health hazards and also cause serious diseases which may affect human life and cause severe damage to their health.

The plant protein, which is highly toxic named as lectin this is dangerous for health and cause serious damage. Gluten is a by-product of lectin and it is also harmful for health. The lectin and its by-product gluten cause serious damage to health and is proven toxic for human life.

There are variety of other fruits which are lectin free and if they lack lectin than they automatically lack gluten. These lectins free and gluten free eatables or foods me include grains, wheat. These are free from lectin and as they are lectin free, so they also lack gluten. These two products are not found in them and they are considered good for health and they are categorized as one of the healthy foods. These are healthy foods and are proved beneficial for health.

So, we can add grains and wheat to our daily routine diet. In this way, we can avoid from the intake of lectin and gluten which are health hazardous. There are other products which are gluten free and are 7also free from lectin, they may include fresh fruits, vegetables, corn, dairy products such as milk, butter, yogurt and all other dairy products. Dairy products may also include fresh cream. These food products must be included in the daily routine diet and must be a part of our diet so we will remain healthy and active all the day. These food products provide energy to our body in real sense and make our bodies more active and fresher.

Are Lectins Really a Problem?

Lectins are a giant class of proteins that exist in the food offer but are mostly common in grains and legumes. The lectins in food bind to carbohydrates, forming glycoproteins. These glycoproteins make some functions in the body, from modifiable the immune system to keeping protein levels within the blood under control.

Yet, consuming too many lectins will also have

contrary effects on health, with some research showing that they may reason contrary symptoms like vomiting and diarrhea and can contribute to leaky gut and could cause changes in immune system.

Luckily, there are various ways to cut back the lectin content of your food without happening a lectin-free diet or severely limiting your eating altogether. Cooking, soaking and sprouting and fermenting your foods can bog down on lectin concentration to promote higher health.

So, the question is "Are lectins extremely bad for you?", Whereas it's true that eating too many foods with lectins have negative effects on health, lectins conjointly play some important roles inside the body. They optimize cell adhesion and are concerned in immune function and the synthesis of glycoproteins.

Lectins are also concerned in immune regulation, and some investigation indicates that they'll have antimicrobial characteristics also. In truth, they have been shown to be actual against many types of bacteria, as well as the strain that reasons staph infections and E. coli. Lectins can also additionally help fight off fungi and viral infections, with in vitro trials signifying that they'll help block the growth of the particular fungus responsible for yeast infections.

It was also noted that the shellfish also proves beneficial for life. It was proved that consumption of shellfish is more beneficial and healthier than other proteins. Shellfish intake is more beneficial and important to human health than the consumption of another animals' protein. Shellfish protein is healthier and more beneficial to human health and life.

Lectin produces more harmful gut bacteria and lead to severe health diseases. More intake of lectin produces a large number of gut bacteria. Gluten is also less beneficial to health and it also produces a harmful bacterium in human gut and that bacteria will cause severe damage to health in future.

And in case if someone avoids wheat, barley, rye, and whole grain from their diet or skip them from their daily routine life, then it may also become one of the causes of producing a gut bacterium and cause severe diseases and severe damage to health.

The use of lectin must be avoided as well because it also inhibits and stops the transmission between body cells and also affect their working.

As we all are aware of the fact that changing eating habits and being addicted or become used to the new eating and diet routine is really a tough job and it really takes time to adopt new routine and to cope up with such routine because everyone is of different nature and have different attitude, everyone has his own digesting abilities and stomach capacity. So, they deal according to their capacities.

Plus, as a result of lectins are involved within the regulation of the immune system, some proof -including a study out of Colorado State University's

Department of Health and Exercise Science revealed within the British Journal of Nutrition - shows that they could conjointly play a role in autoimmune conditions, like rheumatoid arthritis. Autoimmune conditions are a result of the immune system attacking healthy cells within the body, resulting in symptoms like inflammation, fatigue and chronic pain.

Additionally, consuming too several lectins will moreover reason more immediate negative aspect and effects also, as well as digestive problems. Eating uncooked beans, as an example, can cause lectin poisoning and gastroenteritis, a state that reasons symptoms like nausea, vomiting, cramps and diarrhea.

Signs to Many Lectins

The intake of harmful foods other than these may introduce a variety of inflammatory diseases in our body. These variety of inflammatory diseases may include following diseases, such as:

- Serious health problems
- Serious heart diseases
- Stomach issues
- Intestinal inflammation
- Lower abdomen problems
- Diarrhea
- Constipation
- Infant problems

Affect infant's growth and became the cause of slow growth in infants

Also cause variety of mental problems as well, most of the mental issues are being associated with intake of less nutritive food or the intake of such food which may include lectin and gluten because these two products are more dangerous for health and cause severe damage to mental and physical health

It may also lead to cancer, it can be bone marrow cancer, blood cancer, brain tumor or any other type of cancer, in other words, it is also the cause of one the major dangerous and life-threatening disease known as cancer. Cancer is one of the leading causes of death worldwide and it can also be caused because of poor and improper diet and such food products or food items which can be proved health hazardous or such food products which may include lectin or gluten in it because these two products are being proved much harmful for human life and human health.

- Wright loss issues

- Parkinson's disease

- Neurological disorders, improper intake of intake or consumption of lectin and gluten rich products may also lead to serious health problems and affect our neurons as well.

- They are also one of the causes of autoimmune diseases.

Western diet is far better than our Eastern diet. Western diet is also much healthier than our Eastern diet. Western diet may include healthy fruits and vegetables in their diet and are far better than Easter diet. Western people are also safe from many of the hazardous diseased as described earlier. The list of diseases which may cause from the intake of nutrition free food or lectin and gluten rich food. These types of foods may cause a number of or a variety of hazardous diseases and it can be proved life threatening in most of the cases. And also prove vital for health. It causes many deaths in Eastern area because of this nutrition lacking food.

Western diet may include following food items in their diet. These food items may include the following food products, such as:

- Meat, chicken, beef and other type of meat products

- Fresh vegetables

- Fresh fruits

- Fats

- Sugar

- Grains

- Beans

- Legumes

The population of Western area is Long lived as compared to Eastern population. It is being noted that the persons living in west have a long-life span as compared to people living in East. The main reason being the long ages of the West Pakistan people is the consumption of legumes. They add legumes to their diet on regular basis. Legumes is one of the best and nutrition rich product which has to be included in the diet regularly to avoid different problems and to stay away from diseases and also to increase the life span.

Western people also consume beans on large scale. Beans are also proved much beneficial to human health. It helps a person to remain active the entire day, mentally and physically healthy. They consume beans on large scale that's why there is comparatively large life span. The people living in the west live more than Eastern people just because of their food. They intake healthy food and avoid from the junk food, fast food and unhealthy food. They also avoid from the food which is lectin and gluten rich products because they are harmful for health and life.

What is Plant basedDiet diet?

Lectins are the enemy of the Plant basedDiet diet. These are a kind of protein found in plants that scientists believe are part of the defense mechanism plants use to paralyze predatory insects. Lectins go through your body while not being digested and are categorized an anti-nutrient since they lower your ability to soak up key vitamins and minerals. The Plant basedDiet diet calls for avoiding lectins by cutting out an extended list of foods, as well as nightshades (suppose: eggplants, tomatoes, red peppers), out-of-season fruits, grains,and raw legumes, to reportedly cut back inflammation, repair gut health, and prevent weight gain.

The use of lectin must be avoided as well because it also inhibits and stops the transmission between body cells and also affect their working.

As we all are aware of the fact that changing eating habits and being addicted or become used to the new eating and diet routine is really a tough job and it really takes time to adopt new routine and to cope up with such routine because everyone is of different nature and have different attitude, everyone has his own digesting abilities and stomach capacity. So, they deal according to their capacities.

There are variety of foods and drinks for the Plant basedDiet diet. These may include the following salads and drinks.

Chapter 2:
Recipes for Breakfast

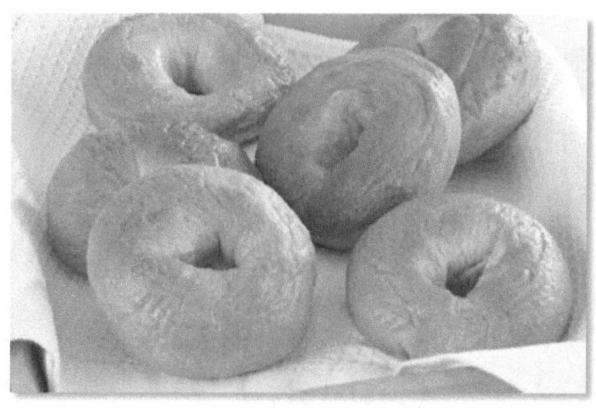

Lectin Free Beigel (Special for Breakfast)

Lectin Free Beigel

A mini bagel for Plant basedDiet may be a low-fat food that may become the bottom for a healthy meal, snack or dessert. Much smaller than an ancient bagel, mini bagels are a healthy option if you are watching your weight and countingcalories.

Ingredients:

- Teaspoons plus 1/4 teaspoon iodized sea salt

- Cups blanched almond flour

- 1 cup tapioca starch (plus additional for boiled water)

- 2 teaspoons bakingpowder

- 2 tablespoons monk fruit sweetener (use a spice grinder to make into powder) or 1 packet stevia

- 2 tablespoons white wine vinegar or champagne

- 1 omega-3 or pastured egg or vegan egg replacer

- Toppings of choice (suggestions: trader joe's "everything but the bagel," caraway seeds, herbs de Provence, or rosemary and sea salt)

Instructions:

Plant basedDiet mini-bagel making is pretty involved, but the end result is so delicious!

- Preheat the oven to 400 degrees F. Place parchment paper on a baking sheet and set aside.

- Fill a 10-inch pot with about 5 inches of water and add the quarter teaspoon of salt. Slowly bring water to a boil.

- In a medium bowl, mix the almond flour, tapioca starch, the remaining salt, baking powder, and monk-fruit powder.

- Before water is at a full boil, remove half a cup and set aside.

- Add the half cup of warm water and the vinegar to the dry mix. If the dough is too sticky, sprinkle lightly with more tapioca starch. If it's too dry, add a little more water.

- Divide the dough into small balls on the baking sheet. You should have about 11-12 mini-bagels.

- Flatten each ball with your hand and mold into the shape of a bagel. Use a utensil or your finger to make a small hole in the center of each. Each finished bagel should be about two and a quarter inches in diameter.

- In groups of 3 or 4, carefully place the bagels in the boiling water.

- Using a strainer, remove them from the water once they float to the top, or after about 1 minute. Place the bagels onto the baking sheet.

- After boiling, bake the bagels for 10 minutes. While they are baking, put the egg in a small bowl and Mix.

- Remove the bagels from the oven and brush each one with the beaten egg, adding your desired toppings before moving onto the next bagel. (This prevents the egg from drying before the toppings adhere.)

- Return bagels to oven and bake for an additional 10 minutes. Increase temperature to 425 degrees F, and bake for another 5-10 minutes, or until the bottoms of the bagels are just golden.

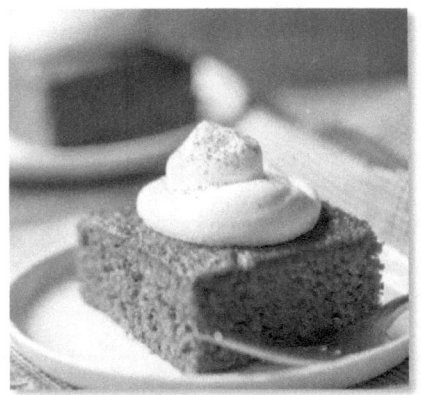

Noreen's Gingerbread Recipe (Hot Favorite)

Noreen's Gingerbread

Nothing says fairy tale Christmas like warm gingerbread, fresh out of the oven. The smell alone is enough to make the grinchiest woman (or man) in the house spontaneously sing Burl Ives.

Unfortunately, real gingerbread with heaping spoonsful of molasses, isn't an option for us lectin-enlightened folk. It's not that we're grinches–we want to enjoy the holidays, preferably pain free. Which may mean saying no to some of our traditional sugary treats.

Ingredients:

- 1 tablespoon softened butter

- 1 tablespoon flour of coconut

- 1 tablespoon tigernut or cassava flour

- 1/2 teaspoon ginger

- 1/4 teaspoon cinnamon

- pinch each of allspice, cloves, and nutmeg

- 1/2 teaspoon baking powder

- teaspoons maple-flavored erythritol syrup

- 1/2 teaspoon apple cider vinegar

- 1/2 tablespoon water

- 1 egg, lightly beaten

Instruction:

- Beat together the butter, coconut flour, tigernut flour, ginger, cinnamon, allspice, and baking powder in a microwave-safe mug.

- Mix in the syrup, cider vinegar, and egg, and beat vigorously with a fork until batter is smooth and consistent (be sure to scrap the sides and bottom of the mug to incorporate all the batter).

- Microwave for 1 1/2 minutes. Scrape around the edges of the mug with a knife, and then shake the muffin out onto a plate. Top with butter and cinnamon.

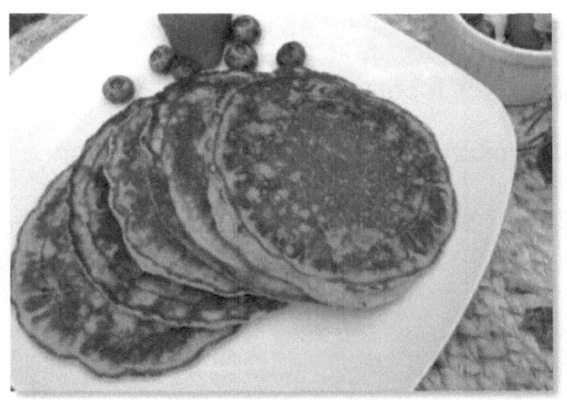

Jimmy's Pancakes with Honey

Jimmy's Pancakes with Honey

Ingredients:

- 1 cup cassava flour

- tablespoons monk's fruit sweetener

- 1 tablespoon baking powder

- 1 teaspoon cinnamon plus more for serving

- 1/4 teaspoon sea salt

- 1/8 teaspoon nutmeg

- 1 1/4 cup goat's milk kefir or coconut/almond yogurt, room temperature

- 1/2 teaspoon vanilla extract

- 3 tablespoons of Honey

- large eggs room temperature

- tablespoons melted butter plus more   for serving

- 1/4 cup water

Instructions:

- Preheat a nonstick griddle to medium-low heat.

- Mix together the flour, baking powder, cinnamon, sea salt sweetener, and nutmeg in a medium sized bowl until mixed well. Mix together the kefir/yogurt, vanilla, eggs, and water in a large bowl until well mix. Mix the butter into the kefir mixture.

- Mix the dry mixture and the wet mixture in the large bowl, Mixing until smooth and well mix.

- Use a 1/4 cup measuring cup to pour batter on the hot griddle, 1-3 pancakes at a time. Cook until bubbles disruption the surface and the undersides are golden brown, about 2 minutes. Flip with a spatula and cook about 1 minute more. Repeat with the remaining batter.

- Serve hot to a warm oven and cover with a slightly damp towel to keep warm. Garnish with cinnamon and serve with butter.

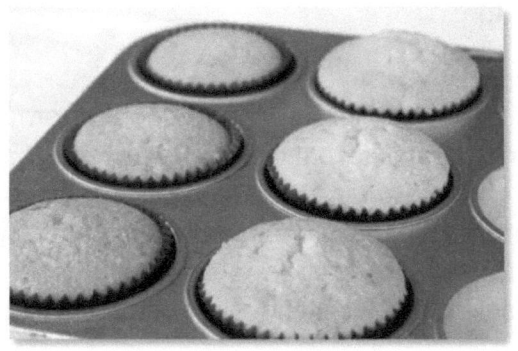

Mexican Vanilla Cupcakes Muffins

Mexican Vanilla Cupcakes

Ingredients:

- 2 tablespoons olive oil
- 1 tablespoon coconut flour
- 1 tablespoon tigernut flour
- teaspoons monk's fruit sweetener
- 1/2 teaspoon vanilla extract
- 1/2 teaspoon baking powder
- pinch of sea salt
- 1 egg, lightly beaten
- Small handful of seasonal fruit or dark chocolate chips (optional)
- To make a chocolate version, add 1/2 tablespoon cocoa powder

Instruction:

• Mix the olive oil, coconut flour, tigernut flour, sweetener, vanilla, baking powder, and salt in a microwave-safe mug. Add the egg, and whip with a fork until texture is smooth and consistent, with no lumps. Be sure to scrape the sides and bottom of the mug. Fold in the fruit or chocolate chips, if using.

• Microwave for 1 minute and 30 seconds. Let cool for a couple minutes, then shake out onto a plate. Serve plain or with butter, honey, or whatever topping you prefer.

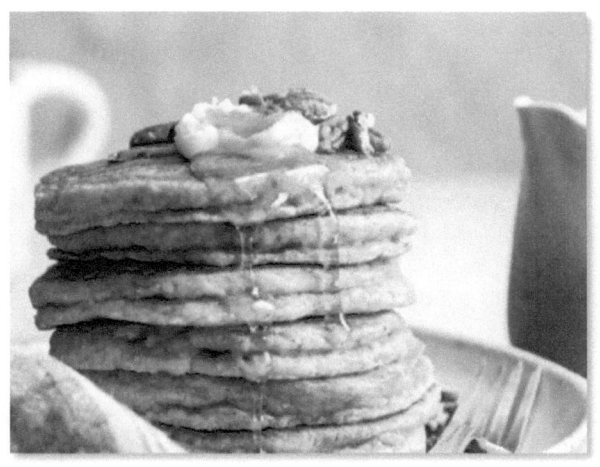

Asma's Peach Honey Pancakes Lectin Free

Asma's Peach Honey Pancakes Lectin Free

Ingredients:

- large omega-3 or pastured eggs

- 1 teaspoon vanilla extract

- 5 drops liquid stevia

- 5 ounces goat's milk kefir

- 1 tablespoon coconut oil, melted

- 1/4 cup coconut flour

- 1/4 cup tapioca flour

- 1/4 cup cassava flour

- 1/4 teaspoon sea salt

- 1/2 teaspoon baking powder

- 1/4 teaspoon baking soda

- ripe peaches, peeled and cut into thin slices

- cinnamon for sprinkling

Instructions:

- Preheat the oven to 350 degrees f. Oil an 8- inch pie pan with coconut oil.

- Beat together the eggs, vanilla, stevia, and kefir. Slowly add the coconut oil, Mixing constantly, so the oil doesn't solidify.

- Add the coconut flour, tapioca flour, cassava flour, sea salt, baking powder, and baking soda. Mix together until batter is smooth.

- Pour the batter into the pie pan. Place half of the peach slices on top of the batter in a single layer. Sprinkle with cinnamon.

- Bake for 30 minutes, testing with a toothpick until it comes out clean. Let the pancake cool to room temperature before slicing. Serve topped with remaining peach slices.

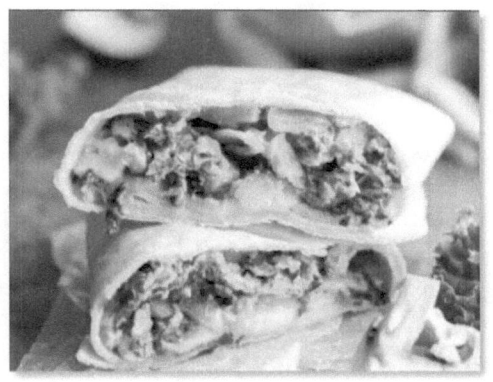

Mexican Burritos with Vegies and Cheese

Mexican Burritos with Vegies and Cheese

Ingredients:

- tablespoons extra-virgin olive oil

- ounces spinach, chopped

- 2 cloves garlic, thinly sliced

- Himalayan sea salt and black pepper

- 6 eggs, beaten

- ounces goat cheese, crumbled

- (8) 6-8-inch cassava flour tortillas

Instructions:

- Heat the oil in a large skillet over medium heat.

- Add the spinach, garlic, 1/2 tsp salt, and 1/4 tsp pepper and cook until spinach is wilted, 2-3 minutes. Spread evenly across the pan.

- Pour the eggs over the spinach and garlic, and let them rest for 30 seconds. Then "bulldoze" the eggs around the pan with a spatula until set, 3-4 minutes.

- Turn off the heat and spread the goat cheese over top of the eggs–let it soften.

- Meanwhile, heat the tortillas in the microwave, covered by a damp paper towel. Heat 4 at a time, for 30 seconds each.

- Spoon eggs into the center of each tortilla, then fold like a taco and serve.

Cupcakes Muffins with Carrots and Dry Fruits

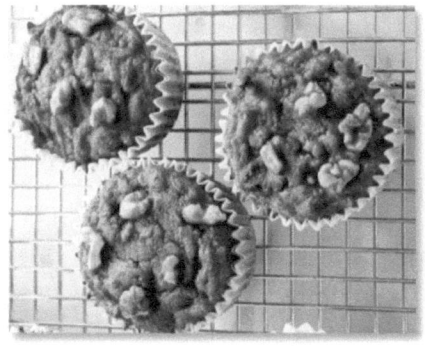

Cupcakes Muffins with Carrots and Dry Fruits

Ingredients:

- 1 1/4 cups blanched almond flour

- 2 tablespoons coconut flour

- 1/2 teaspoon baking soda

- 1/8 teaspoon salt

- 1 1/2 teaspoons Pulver cinnamon

- 1/2 teaspoon Pulver ginger

- 1/4 teaspoon Pulver nutmeg

- Two omega-3 or pastor and eggs or Vegan Eggs

- 1/3 cup MCT oil or avocado oil

- 2/3 cup vapid coconut milk

- 1/3 cup Swerve (erythritol)

- 2 teaspoons vanilla

- Dry Fruits

- Two large carrots, grated

- 1/4 chopped walnuts

Instructions:

- Preheat the oven to 350°F. Prepare the muffin tin with cupcake liners and set aside.

- In a large bowl, mix together the coconut flour, baking soda almond flour, cinnamon, ginger, and nutmeg.

- In a small bowl, mix the eggs, oil, coconut milk, Swerve, and vanilla.

- Mix what ingredients into dry, then add the grated carrots and walnuts.

- Fold to mix.

- Portion into the muffin tin, dividing every mixture evenly among 12 cups.

- Bake for 12 to 18 minutes, or until a toothpick inserted into the center of the muffins comes out clean. Allow my friends to cool slightly before serving. When stored in an airtight container, muffins will stay fresh five days in the refrigerator or three months in the freezer.

Muffin in a Mug (Coconut and Almond Flour)

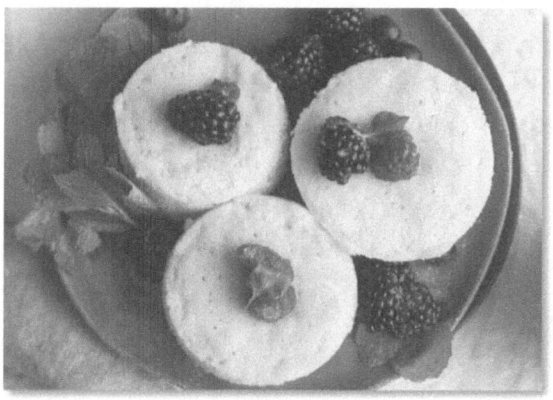

Muffin in a Mug (Coconut and Almond Flour)

Ingredients:

- 1 tablespoon melted coconut oil

- 1 tablespoon macadamia nut oil or olive-oil

- 2 tablespoon coconut flour and almond flour

- 1/2 teaspoon aluminum-free baking powder

- 1 pinch of iodized salt

- 2 teaspoons of common sugar

- 3 teaspoons of water

- 1 large pastured or omega-3 egg, lightly beaten

Instruction:

Place the ingredients in an eight to twelve-ounce microwave-safe mug, mixing well with a fork or spatula. Be sure to scrape the bottom and sides. Let it sit for a few seconds. Microwave on high for one minute and twenty-thirty Seconds. Using a pot holder, remove the mug from the microwave and invert, shaking out the muffin. Let cool for a couple of minutes before eating.

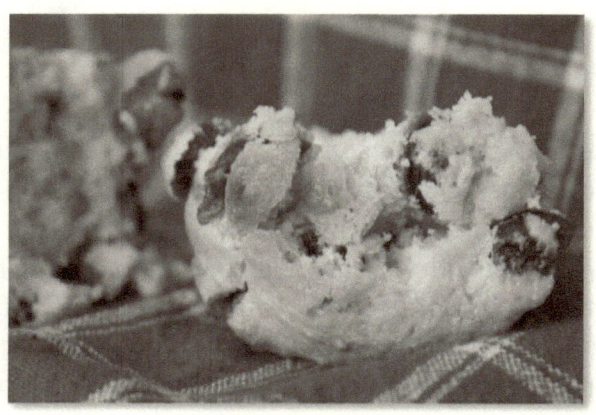

American Muffins Orange Flavored

American Muffins Orange Flavored

Ingredients:

- 1/4 cup coconut flour

- 1/4 teaspoon iodized salt

- 1/4 teaspoon of baking soda

- 1/4 cup melted coconut oil

- 1/4 cup Just Like Sugar or xylitol

- 3 large pastured or omega-3 eggs

- 3 teaspoon of orange zest

- 1/2 cup dried, unsweetened cranberries

Instructions:

Heat the oven to 350°F. Line a normal half dozen-cup muffin tin with paper liners. Place coconut flour, salt, and baking soda in a very food processor with a blade. Add the coconut, Just Like Sugar, eggs, and orange zest. Pulse until blended. Remove the processor blade and stir in the cranberries by hand. Scoop the batter into the muffin tins, filling to merely beneath the rim. Bake for twenty minutes. Let cool on a rack for fifteen minutes before serving.

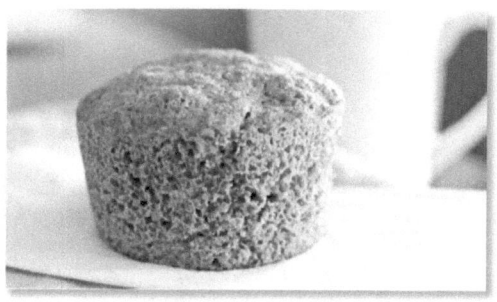

Cinnamon flavored Muffins

Cinnamon Flavored Muffins

Ingredients:

- 1/4 cup Pulverflaxseed

- 1/3 tablespoon cinnamon

- 1 large pastured or omega-3 egg

- 3 teaspoons melted coconut oil

- 1 teaspoon aluminum-free baking powder

- 1 packet stevia

Instructions:

Place all the ingredients in an 8 to twelve-ounce microwave-safe mug, and combine well with a fork or spatula. Be sure to scrape the bottom and sides. Let it sit for a few seconds. Microwave on high for one minute. Check and cook for one more five to 15 second if the muffin appears still wet in the middle.

Using a pot holder, take away the mug from the microwave and invert, shaking out the muffin. Let cool for two minutes before eating. Enjoy your meal!

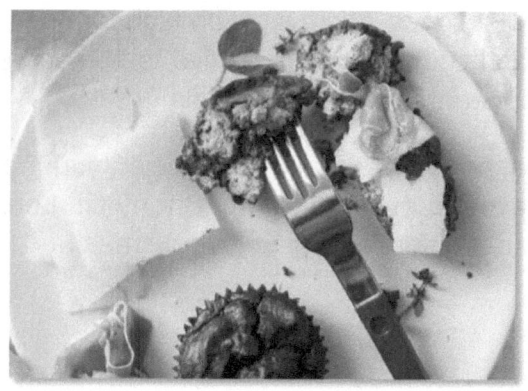

Green Vegies Muffins

Green Vegies Muffins

Ingredients:

- One Pound of Turkey Chorizo

- One 10-ounce chopped kale

- 3 omega eggs

- 6 teaspoons perilla oil

- 2 cloves garlic, peeled, or 1 teaspoon garlic powder

- 6 teaspoons of Italian seasoning

- 6 teaspoons of dried minced onion

- 1/2 teaspoon sea salt, preferably iodized

- 1/2 teaspoon cracked black pepper

Instructions:

1. Set the oven to 350°F. Line a medium cup muffin tin with paper liners. Put in a non- Teflon frying pan. Cook at medium heat, moving often, until browned, around 7 to 11 minutes.

• Use a knife to make small holes in the bag, Place in the microwave on high heat for 2 and half minutes. Cut a tiny edge off the corner of the bag, and press as much water out of the bag as much as you can.

• Place the drained spinach, olive oil, garlic, eggs, Italian seasoning, salt, pepper, and onion in a super speed blender until thoroughly mixed. Transfer to a large bowl and stir in the sausage until well mixed.

• Fill the muffin tins to the rim. Bake for 25 to 33 minutes, until the tops start to brown. Place out from the oven and make them cool before removing individual muffins.

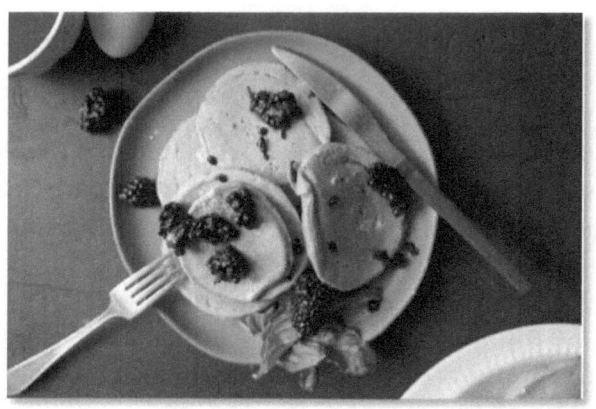

Hamzi's Plant basedDiet Pancakes

Hamzi's Plant basedDiet Pancakes

Ingredients:

- Peeling raw green plantains

- 4 omega-3 eggs

- 1/2 tablespoon vanilla extract

- 6 teaspoons melted coconut oil

- 2 tablespoon sugar

- A pinch of iodized salt

- 1/2 teaspoon of baking soda

Instructions:

Place the plantain pieces in a blender or food processor and purée. You ought to have concerning two cups. Add the eggs and mix to create a sleek batter. Add the vanilla extract, 3 tablespoons of melted coconut oil, Just Like Sugar, the salt, and baking soda. Process on high for 2 to 3 minutes, till sleek.

Heat 3 teaspoons coconut oil in an exceedingly pan. When the oil shimmers, one pair of cups live with batter and pour into the pan. Repeat for two to three more pancakes. Cook 4 to five minutes, till the high appearance fairly dry and has little bubbles. Flip and cook 1 1/2 to two minutes additional. Repeat with remaining batter, adding a lot of oil as required.

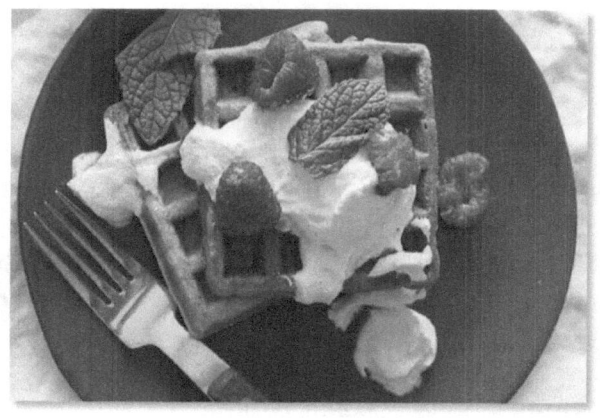

Waffles with Cream and Strawberries

Waffles with Cream and Strawberries

Ingredients:

- 4 omega-3 eggs

- 2 tablespoons Vital Proteins marine collagen

- Half cup cassava flour

- Half cup melted coconut oil

- 3 teaspoon local honey

- 2 Pinches of Baking soda

- 4 Strawberries

- A pinch of salt

Instructions:

- Heat a waffle iron device. Put the eggs, marine collagen, if you need, cassava flour, coconut oil, honey, baking soda, and salt in a super speed blender to mix well on high for 45 seconds or until well mixed.

- If serving as a dessert, you may want to sprinkle a light coating of Just like Sugar and place 1/4 cup wild blueberries on top of each waffle for garnishing and awesome flavor. But always reminisce, it is best to retreat from sweet!

Chapter 3:

Beverages & Salads

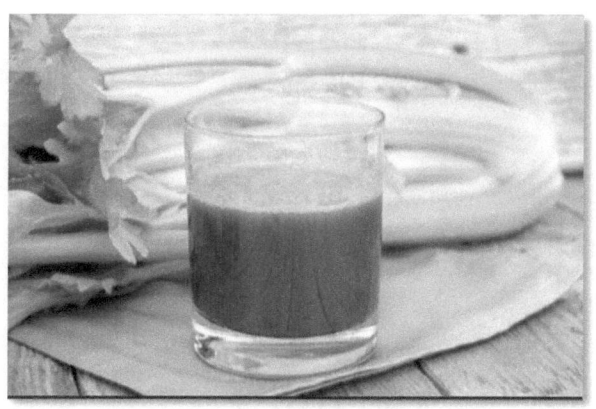

Mustard Plant Juice

Mustard Plant Juice

Ingredients:

- Grab two bunches of mustard plant.

- Cut off the base and the top of the stalks.

- Wash them gently in a colander.

- Feed the celery through the feeding tube of your juicer.

- Serve the juice immediately and keep any leftovers in a tightly sealed jar in the fridge.

Instructions:

• Grab two bunches of Mustard Plant and cut off the base and the top of the stalks.

• Wash them gently in a colander.

• Chop the celery stalks into thirds and place them in the base of your high-speed blender.

• Add 1/4 cup of water and put the lid on the blender. Blend until smooth, using the tamper to push the celery into the blades if necessary.

• Place a clean nut milk bag over the mouth of a pitcher and pour the blended celery through the nut milk bag. Use your hands to squeeze the celery juice through the bag.

• Serve the juice immediately and keep any leftovers in a tightly sealed jar in the fridge.

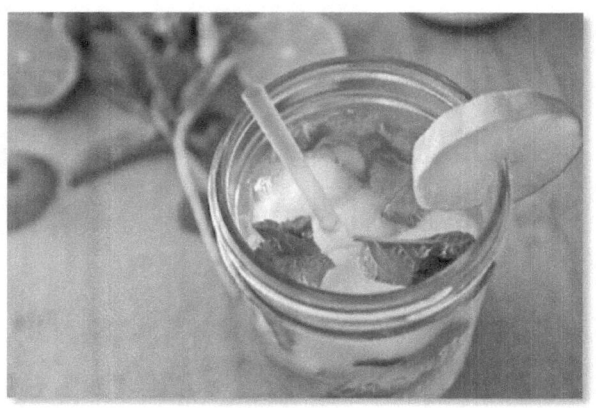

Fresh Vinegar Drink

Fresh Vinegar Drink

Diet Coke, Diet Pepsi, Diet Dr. Pepper, Diet Root Beer, or diet whatever kills your gut buddies, but my surefire replacement is the color of your previous cola and is equally fizzy. The balsamic vinegar contains resveratrol, one of the most powerful polyphenol compounds, which will wonder for you-and also the inner you.

Napa Valley Naturals Grand Reserve is my favorite balsamic vinegar, for its thick consistency and terribly sleek depth of flavor. Once you've tried this drink, you'll never go back to cola!

Ingredients:

- 8 to 10 ounces of high-pH carbonated chilled water
- 6 teaspoons Traditional balsamic vinegar

Instruction:

Mix the carbonated chilled water and balsamic in a regular sized glass, shake, and enjoy this life-giving fresh fountain drink!

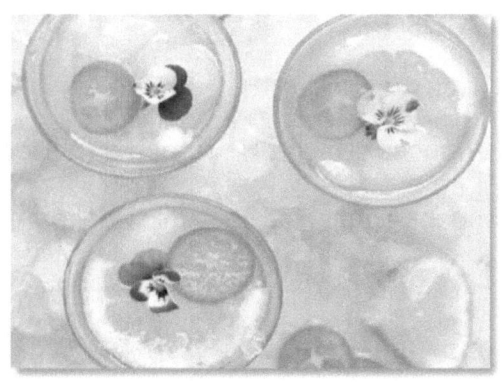

Awesome Pear Lemon Drink

Awesome Pear Lemon Drink

Ingredients:

- 2 Lemons

- A pinch of Salt

- A pinch of Sugar

- 1 Pear

Instructions:

- Peel and chop a pear.

- Juice lemons using this juicer or your own. If you microwave the lemon 10 seconds before juicing, you'll get maximum juice.

- Add the pear, lemon juice and water to a high- speed blender and blend until the liquid is completely blended.

- Put the lemonade in the refrigerator to completely chill through.

- Serve with ice.

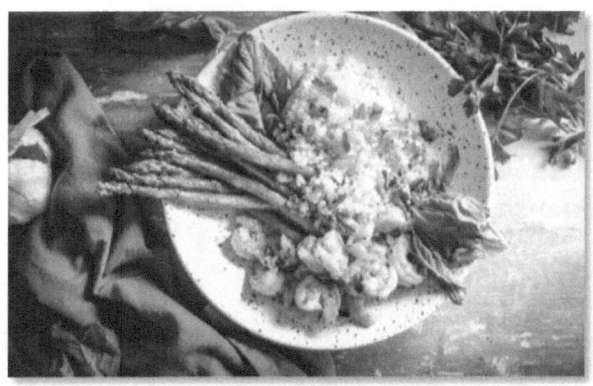

Shrimp with Green Salad

Shrimps with Green Salad

Ingredients:

- 1/2 cup extra-virgin olive oil plus more for brushing

- 4 strips lemon zest

- Cloves garlic sliced

- 1 pinch red pepper

- Sea salt

- 1 pound wild-caught jumbo shrimp shells on

- 1/2 cup chopped fresh parsley

- 5 ounces mixed greens

- White wine vinegar for sprinkling

Instructions:

•   Heat the oil, lemon zest, garlic, red pepper, and ¼ teaspoon salt in a small pot over medium heat until it sizzles, 2-3 minutes.

•   Preheat a large skillet over medium heat, and brush with a little olive oil. Place the shrimp in the skillet and cook, covered, without moving them, until opaque throughout, 3-5 minutes.

•   Transfer to a large bowl. Add the lemon oil and parsley and toss to mix. Divide the greens among 4 plates, and top with the shrimp. Drizzle the extra dressing at the bottom of the bowl over the greens. Sprinkle with white wine vinegar.

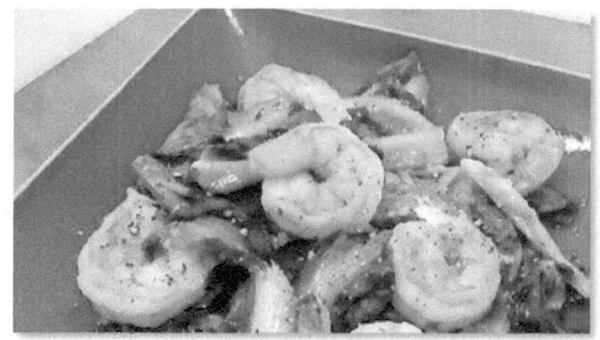

Shrimp with Endive Salad

Shrimp with Endive Salad

Toss together:

- 1-pound well-cooked shrimps

- 1 head escarole

- 1/2 red onion, sliced

- 1 bunch radishes, quartered

Caper-Herb Vinaigrette

Mix together:

- 1 small shallot, finely chopped
- 6 teaspoons capers
- Two Cloves
- 6 teaspoons chopped fresh chives
- 1/3 tablespoon of Dijon mustard
- 6 teaspoons of white wine vinegar
- 2 tablespoons of olive oil
- A pinch of Salt and pepper

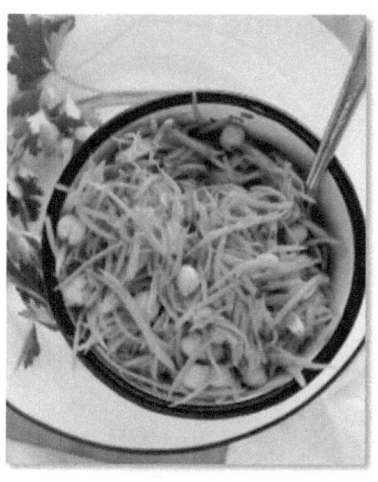

Fresh Carrot Salad with Honey

Fresh Carrot Salad with Honey

Ingredients:

- ½ pound carrots, peeled

- ¼ cup purple cabbage, sliced very thinly

- Handful of bean sprouts

- 2 Tbsp. chopped fresh parsley

- 1 tablespoon raw apple cider vinegar

- 1 Tsp. flax oil

- Sea salt, to taste

- Freshly ground black pepper, to taste

Instructions:

- Grate the carrots in a food processor. Set aside. Prepare rest of the ingredients.

- In a medium bowl, combine the carrots, cabbage, bean sprouts and parsley.

- Pour the ACV over the ingredients and lastly massage the flax oil into the salad with freshly washed hands.

- Season to taste with the option of adding salt/pepper.

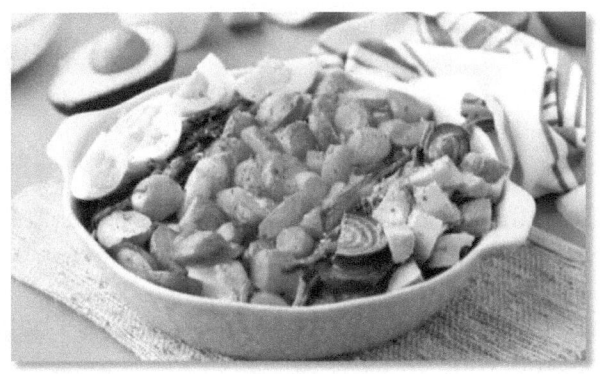

Roasted Cobb Salad

Roasted Cobb Salad

Serve each component in heaping mounds on a serving platter:

- cooked, diced chicken

- roasted romaine hearts, chopped

- 2 hard-boiled eggs, sliced

- 1 bunch scallions, chopped

- 2 large, ripe avocados, sliced

- ounces goat cheese, crumbled

Adobo Cream Dressing

Mix together:

- 1/2 cup sour cream

- 1/4 cup heavy cream

- juice of 1 lime

- 1 tablespoon red wine vinegar

- 1 tablespoon adobo sauce from canned chipotles

- 1 teaspoon salt

- 1 teaspoon cumin

Instructions:

Preheat an oven to 450 degrees F. Brush 2 pastured chicken breast halves (boneless, skinless) and 3 large hearts of romaine (halved lengthwise) with olive oil. Season with chili powder, cumin, salt, and pepper. Bake chicken alone on a parchment lined baking sheet for 10 minutes. Arrange the romaine, cut side down, around the chicken and bake for another 5-10 minutes, until the lettuce is browned at the edges and the chicken is cooked through.

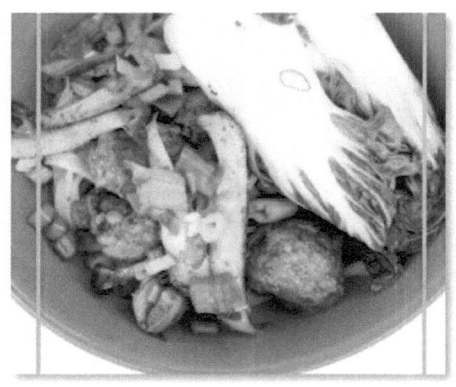

Meatball & Bok Choy Salad

Meatball & Bok Choy Salad

Toss together:

- Cooked meatballs

- Heads baby bok choy, chopped (alternatively, serve each salad bowl an individual bok choy)

- Sautéed shiitake mushrooms

- 4 scallions, thinly sliced

- 1/2 cup chopped fresh cilantro

- 1/4 cup chopped salted macadamia nuts

Red Pepper Vinaigrette Mix together:

- 3 tablespoons lime juice

- 1 tablespoon coconut aminos

- 2 teaspoons golden monk fruit sweetener

- 1 tablespoon sesame oil

- 1/2 teaspoon red pepper

Instructions:

Mix 1-pound pastured Pulver pork with 2 cloves chopped garlic, and a liberal sprinkling of salt and pepper. Form mixture into 20 1-inch meatballs. Heat 2 tablespoons oil in a large skillet over medium-high heat. Cook the meatballs, turning occasionally, until browned and cooked through, 8-10 minutes. Remove to a plate, leaving the pan drippings behind. Add 2 cups of sliced shiitake mushrooms to the skillet, and sauté for about 3-5 minutes.

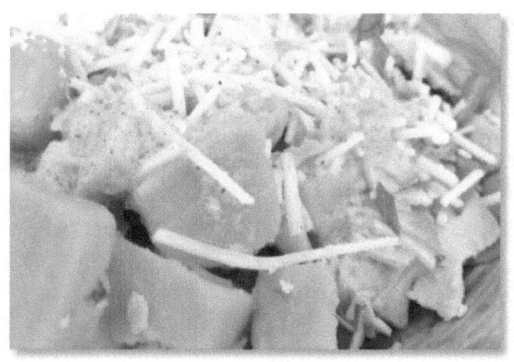

Prosciutto, Sweet Potato, and Arugula Salad

Prosciutto, Sweet Potato, and Arugula Salad

Ingredients:

- 1-pound sweet potato, peeled and cubed
- sea salt and black pepper
- 1/4 cup extra-virgin olive oil
- 1 tablespoon white wine vinegar
- 1 tablespoon Dijon mustard
- ounces baby arugula
- 2 ounces prosciutto di Parma, shredded
- 2 ounces real Swiss cheese, shredded
- 1/4 cup fresh tarragon leaves
- 1/4 cup Parmigiano-Reggiano, shredded

Instructions:

- Place the sweet potatoes in a large pot, cover with cold water, and bring to a boil.

- Add 1 1/2 tablespoons of salt, reduce heat, and simmer until tender, about 12 minutes. Drain, run under cold water, and dice thinner.

- Temporarily, in a small bowl, Mix the oil, vinegar, mustard, 1/2 teaspoon salt, and 1/4 teaspoon pepper.

- Divide the arugula among 4 bowls. Top with prosciutto, swiss cheese, tarragon, and sweet potatoes. Drizzle with the dressing and sprinkle with Parmigiano-Reggiano.

Chapter 4:

Main & Side Dishes

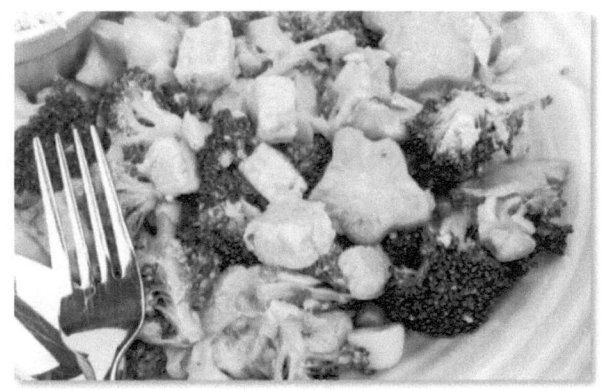

Garlic-Ginger Chicken & Broccoli

Garlic-Ginger Chicken & Broccoli

Ingredients:

- 3/4-pound pastured chicken breast, cubed

- 3 scallion whites, thinly sliced

- 2 cloves garlic, minced and divided

- 1 inch peeled fresh ginger, minced and divided

- 2 tablespoons coconut aminos

- 1 tablespoon golden monk fruit sweetener

- 1 tablespoon arrowroot starch

- Sea salt and black pepper

- 1 tablespoon dry sherry or cooking wine

- 1 tablespoon sesame oil

- 3 tablespoons avocado oil

- 2 broccoli crowns, cut into florets

- 2 broccoli stalks, trimmed and sliced (keep separate from florets)

- Riced cauliflower, shirataki rice, or cooked/cooled/reheated Indian basmati rice, for serving

Instructions:

- Toss the chicken with the scallions, half the garlic and ginger, coconut aminos, sweetener, arrowroot starch, 1 teaspoon salt, dry sherry, and

1 tablespoon sesame oil. Marinate at room temperature for 15 minutes.

- Meanwhile, heat 1 tablespoon avocado oil over high temperature in a big wok. Mix the broccoli stems, and shake-fry for half minute. Mix the florets, the remaining garlic and ginger, half cup water, a pinch of salt, and pepper to taste. Stir-fry until broccoli is bright green and crisp, about 120 seconds. Place into a plate.

- Heat the residual avocado-oil. Mix the chicken and marinade, and stir-fry until chicken is browned, about 3 minutes. Return the broccoli to the pan and toss to mix. Stir in ¼ cup water to thin. Season with salt and pepper and serve over rice.

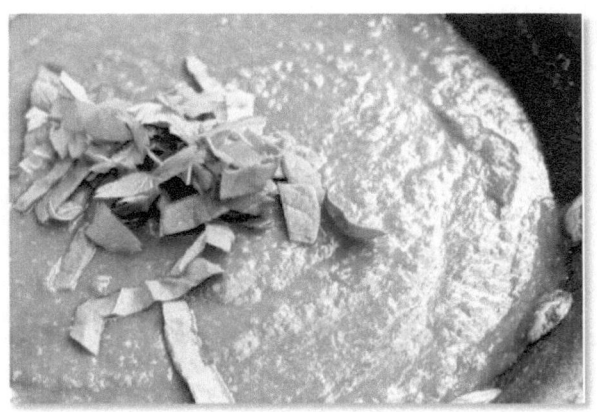

Red Wine & Sweet Potato Marinara

Red Wine & Sweet Potato Marinara

Ingredients:

- 1 15-ounce can sweet potato purée(or homemade–see above)

- 1 cup dry red wine

- 3/4 cup heavy cream or coconut cream (from the top of the can)

- 1/4 cup chopped fresh basil leaves, divided

- 1/4 cup chopped fresh parsley leaves, divided

- 1/4 cup grated Parmigiano-Reggiano

Instructions:

• Heat the sweet potato purée in a large saucepan over medium-high heat. Add half the basil and parsley to the skillet and cook for 2 minutes, stirring constantly. Add the wine and heavy cream/coconut cream.

• Bring to a boil, reduce the heat to medium-low and simmer until the sauce thickens, 7-8 minutes (or longer, if using a thinner heavy cream). Add the parmigiano at the end and stir until melted.

• Serve your lectin-free pasta sauce over your favorite lectin-free noodles or delicious meatballs. Top your dish with the remaining herbs.

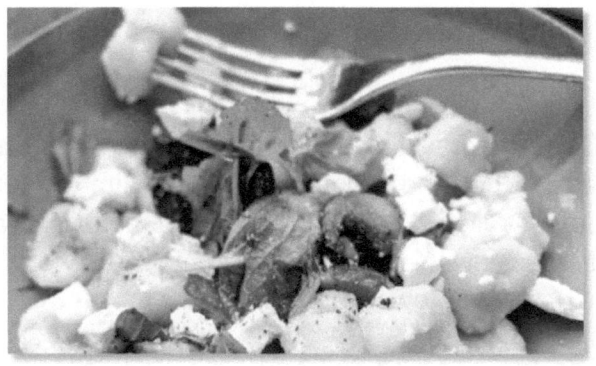

Three-Ingredient Cauliflower Gnocchi

Ingredient Cauliflower Gnocchi

Ingredients:

- 1-pound large pieces of cauliflower florets

- 1.5 – 2 cups cassava flour

- omega-3 egg (1 egg)

- Pinch of Sea Salt and Black Pepper

- 2 tablespoons of olive oil

- 10 ounces chopped bella mushrooms

- Chopped cloves garlic

- 2 ounces of crumbled Greek feta

- Fresh basil leaves for garnishing

Instructions:

• Cover the cauliflower florets with cold water during a massive pot and produce to a boil. Simmer for 15 minutes. Drain, cool slightly, and then mash in a large bowl. Use a towel to squeeze out some of the water and come back cauliflower to the bowl.

• Add the egg and salt and stir to mix. Slowly add the flour, working together with your hands, till the dough now not sticks to the bowl (or your hands), however isn't crumbly. Bring a large pot of water to a boil.

• Roll the dough into long snakes, regarding the width of your thumb. Cut into 1-inch items and press a thumbprint into every piece. Carefully drop the items into the boiling water, operating in two batches. When they float to the surface, remove with a slotted spoon and store in a coated dish to stay heat.

• Meanwhile, heat the oil in an exceedingly massive skillet over medium-high heat. Add the mushrooms, garlic, and several grinds of salt and pepper. Cook, tossing, until just tender, six-eight minutes. Add to the gnocchi and toss to combine. Serve sprinkled with feta, chopped basil, and extra pepper. Drizzle with olive oil.

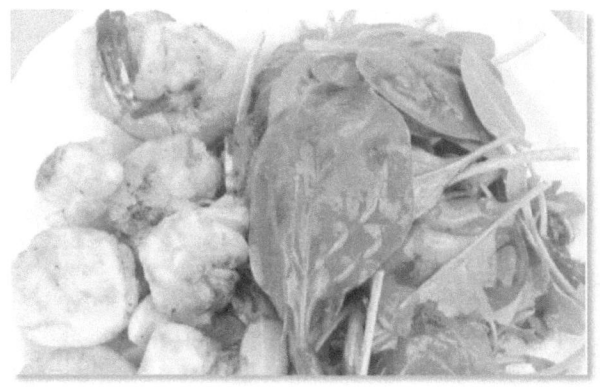

Wild Shrimp with Lemon Oil & Greens

Wild Shrimp with Lemon Oil & Greens

Ingredients:

- 1/2 cup extra-virgin olive oil plus more for brushing

- strips lemon zest

- 2 cloves garlic sliced

- 1 pinch red pepper

- Sea salt

- 1 pound wild-caught jumbo shrimp shells on

- 1/2 cup chopped fresh parsley

- ounces mixed greens

- White wine vinegar for sprinkling

Instructions:

• Heat the oil, lemon zest, garlic, red pepper, and ¼ teaspoon salt in a small pot over medium heat until it sizzles, 2-3 minutes.

• Preheat a large skillet over medium heat, and brush with a little olive oil. Place the shrimp in the skillet and cook, covered, without moving them, until opaque throughout, 3-5 minutes.

• Transfer to a large bowl. Add the lemon oil and parsley and toss to mix. Divide the greens among 4 plates, and top with the shrimp. Drizzle the extra dressing at the bottom of the bowl over the greens. Sprinkle with white wine vinegar.

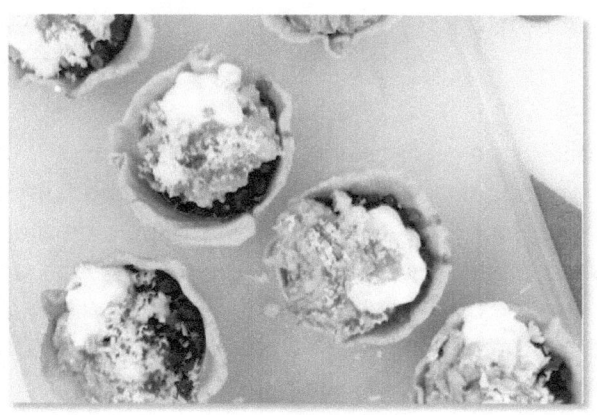

Cassava Flour Taco Cups

Cassava Flour Taco Cups

Ingredients:

- Olive oil, ghee, or avocado oil for greasing pan

- 1 cup cassava flour

- 1/2 cup unsweetened coconut milk, room temperature

- 1/4 cup melted salted butter or palm shortening (add 1/2 teaspoon salt if not salted)

- 1/4 cup warm water

- Instructions

- Preheat oven to 425 degrees f. Oil the undersides of a 12-cup muffin tin.

Instructions:

- Mix the cassava flour, coconut milk, butter/shortening, and warm water in a medium bowl until well mix. Separate dough into approximately 12 1-ounce balls. Lightly sprinkle 2 sides of each dough ball in a little bit of cassava flour. Then roll with a pin or flatten in a tortilla press between 2 pieces of parchment paper into small 4-inch rounds.

- Peel dough away from the parchment paper and drape over the undersides of muffin cups, folding and pressing dough to adhere to cup shape, as necessary. Bake until golden brown, about 20 minutes. Let cool before filling with desired toppings and serving.

- Storage: cups can be sealed and stored at room temperature for up to a week or frozen for up to a month. To reheat, bake at 425 degrees f for 8-10 minutes (they will be crispier than the initial cups).

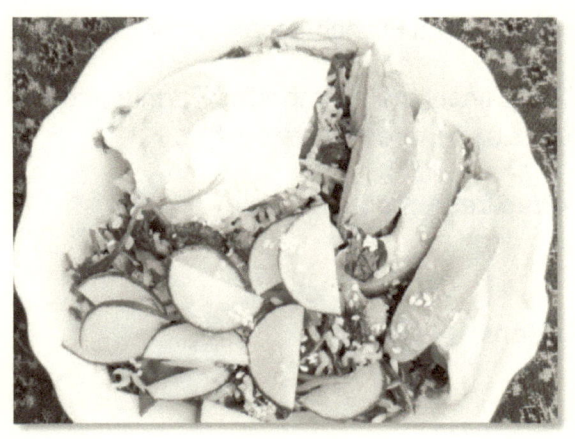

Low Carb Recipes for Shirataki Noodles

Low Carb Recipes for Shirataki Noodles

Ingredients:

- 2 packs angel hair shirataki noodles

- 1 tablespoon olive oil

- 2 cups wild caught seafood broth

- 6 cloves garlic, peeled and crushed

- 1/4 teaspoon red pepper

- sea salt and black pepper

- 24 small hard-shell, wild-caught clams, scrubbed clean

- 4 tablespoons French/Italian butter, cut into cubes

- 1/2 cup finely grated imported Parmigiano-Reggiano, plus more for serving

- 1/4 cup fresh chopped parsley

Instructions:

- Drain and rinse the shirataki noodles with warm water. Boil for 2 minutes and dry out, if desired.

- Heat broiler to high with a rack six inches from the flame. Mix the oil, broth, garlic, red pepper, and a pinch of salt in an exceedingly 9×13-inch glass baking dish. Broil till the garlic is toasted, regarding a pair of minutes. Add the clams, and continue to broil until all the clams have opened, for four minutes.

- Heat a large pot over medium-low heat, and place the noodles in the pot. Add the butter, parmigiano, and parsley, and toss until butter is melted and noodles are coated.

- Remove the clams from the oven, and serve them with the garlic and broth over the noodles. Sprinkle with additional parmigiano and black pepper.

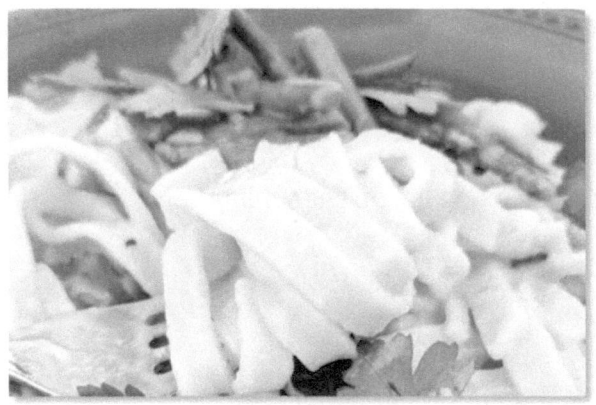

Fettuccine Alfredo with Fresh Spring Vegetables

Fettuccine Alfredo with Fresh Spring Vegetables

Ingredients:

- Sea salt and black pepper

- servings of grain-free pasta (fettuccine or linguine style)

- 1/4 cup extra-virgin olive oil, plus more for tossing

- ounces shiitake mushrooms, sliced

- 1 bunch of trimmed thin asparagus

- 1 cup imported Italian mascarpone

- 1/4 cup grated Parmigiano-Reggiano

- 1/2 cup chopped fresh Italian parsley or basil leaves

- 1/2 teaspoon Italian seasoning

- Zest of 1/2 lemon

Instructions:

- Cook pasta according to package directions. Strain, reserving 1 cup of cooking water and toss with extra-virgin olive oil in a colander.

- Heat 2 tablespoons olive oil in a large skillet over medium heat. Add mushrooms and raise heat to medium-high heat. Cook undisturbed for 1-2 minutes and then cook, stirring, for 2 minutes more. Add the remaining olive oil, the asparagus, and ½ teaspoon salt. Cook, stirring, until asparagus is crisp tender and mushrooms are completely browned, about 3 minutes.

- Turn off heat and add the mascarpone and the cooked noodles. Toss to coat and add the reserved cooking water, ¼ cup at a time, to moisten the noodles and thin the sauce to desired consistency. Gently stir in the pecorino, herbs, Italian seasoning, and lemon zest. Sprinkle with salt and pepper to taste and serve immediately.

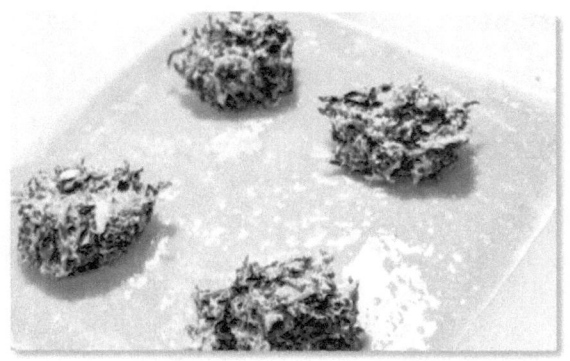

Ravioli with Coconut Wraps

Ravioli with Coconut Wraps

Ingredients:

For Ravioli

- tablespoons extra-virgin olive oil, divided

- 1 10-ounce package frozen, chopped spinach, thawed and squeezed dry

- 1/4 cup imported Italian mascarpone

- 1/4 cup grated Parmigiano-Reggiano

- coconut wraps (square)

- 2 large pastured or omega-3 eggs, beaten with 1 teaspoon water

For Basil pesto

- 2 cups packed fresh basil

- 1/4 cup pine nuts

- 1 ounces Parmigiano-Reggiano, crumbled

- 2 cloves garlic

- 1/2 cup extra-virgin olive oil

- ounces mixed salad greens

- Additional olive oil and balsamic vinegar

Instructions:

- Heat 2 tablespoons olive oil in a large sauté pan. Add the spinach, and cook for 2 minutes. Place in a bowl, and stir in the mascarpone and the parmigiano.

- Line up 2 1/2 wraps on a cutting board. Brush with the egg and water mixture. Use a tablespoon to arrange 4 dollops of filling in each of the 4 corners of the wrap (2 on the 1/2 wrap), leaving an inch or more of space between dollops. Brush another wrap (or 1/2 wrap) with egg wash, and place directly on top, pressing around the filling and sealing the edges. Use a fluted ravioli cutter to cut out 4 squares of ravioli. Alternatively, use a pizza cutter to cut straight-edge square or round raviolis. Keep on the cutting board and cover with a linen towel to rest.

• Make the basil pesto by pulsing all of the ingredients in a blender or food processor until smooth.

• Heat the remaining 2 tablespoons olive oil in the sauté pan over medium heat. Working in batches, fry the ravioli for 2-3 minutes total, flipping halfway through. Serve with pesto and salad greens. Drizzle with additional olive oil and balsamic vinegar.

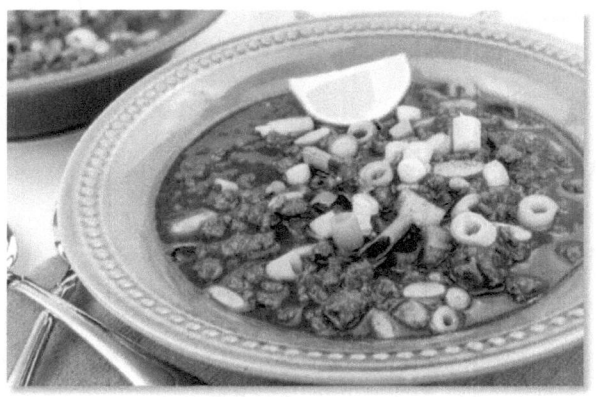

The Best Ever Lectin-Free Chili

The Best Ever Lectin-Free Chili

Ingredients:

- 1/4 cup of avocado oil, divided
- 2 pounds chopped beef
- Pinch of Sea salt and black pepper
- Small pieces of cloves garlic
- 1 medium sized chopped onion
- Ribs celery, finely diced
- 6 teaspoons chili powder
- 1/2 tablespoons Pulver cumin

- 1/4 teaspoon Pulver cinnamon

- Pinch Pulver cloves

- 2 cups grass-fed beef broth

- ounces pine nuts

- 1 15-ounce can sweet potato purée

- 3 teaspoons sauce from preserved chipotles in adobo

- 1/2 tablespoons red wine vinegar

- 1/2 teaspoons coconut aminos

- Sliced scallions and lime wedges, for garnish

- Sour cream, for serving (optional)

Instructions:

- Heat 1 teaspoon oil in an exceedingly massive nonstick skillet over high heat. Add one-pound Pulver beef and ½ teaspoon salt, and brown- breaking the meat apart with a spatula-for 3-4 minutes. Transfer to the instant pot, and repeat with the remaining beef.

- Turn heat down to medium, and warmth the remaining teaspoon oil. Add the garlic, onion, and celery, and cook for five minutes, till soft. Add the chili powder, cumin, cinnamon, and cloves, and stir, cooking for one minute. Pour within the broth, scrape the bottom of the pan, and transfer to the instant pot.

• Add the pine nuts, sweet potato puree, adobo sauce, wine vinegar, coconut aminos, two teaspoons salt, and pepper to style. Cover, and use the slow cook program on medium setting for six hours. Be certain the knob is turned to vent the steam. Serve with scallions, lime wedges, and bitter cream, if desired.

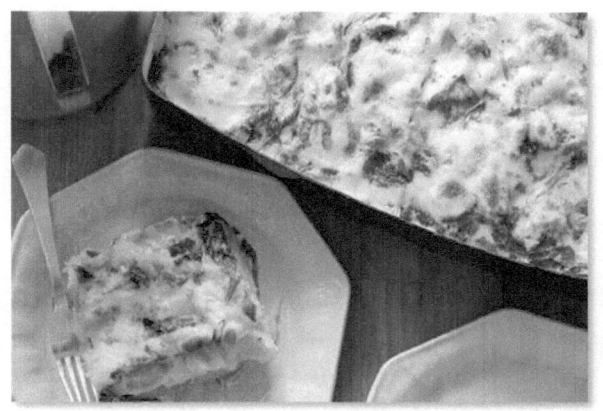

Root Vegetable Lasagna

Root Vegetable Lasagna

Ingredients:

- 1/4 cup olive oil, plus more for baking dish
- 1 yellow onion, diced
- 1 cup diced parsnips
- 1 cup diced celery root
- 1 cup diced rutabaga or turnips
- 1 sprig rosemary, leaves minced
- 2 garlic cloves, peeled and minced

- 1 tsp. Iodized sea salt

- 1/2 tsp. Black pepper

- 1/2 cup water

- 1/2 cup coconut milk

- 2 cups goat's or sheep's milk ricotta or 3 cups coconut yogurt

- 1/2 tsp. Dried oregano

- 1 lemon, zested and juiced

- 1 cup loosely packed basil, julienned

- 2 omega-3 or pastured eggs or vegan eggs

- 1 large sweet potato, thinly sliced (as lasagna noodles; using a mandolin helps)

- 1/2 cup grated Parmigiano-Reggiano

Instructions:

- Preheat the oven to 375°. Spray a 9 × 13-inch baking dish with oil, and set aside.

- First, make your sauce: heat olive oil in a large saucepan over medium-high heat. Add the onion, and cook 2 to 3 minutes, until translucent. Add the parsnips, celery root and rutabaga or turnips, as well as rosemary and garlic, and cook for 15 to 20 minutes, stirring frequently, until vegetables are tender. Add the salt and pepper and blend using an immersion blender (or transfer to a blender), and process until smooth. Sauce should be consistency of thick tomato sauce. If too thick, add water, a little at a time. Mix in coconut milk and set aside.

• In a large bowl, mix the ricotta or coconut yogurt, oregano, lemon zest and juice, basil and the eggs. Set aside.

• Spoon half a cup of the root veggie sauce into the base of your baking dish, and layer on one layer of the thin sliced sweet potato "noodles." Top with half a cup of the ricotta mixture, then repeat until pan is full. (it will take three or four layers.) Sprinkle the top of the lasagna with the Parmigiano-Reggiano, and cover the pan with foil.

• Bake for 35 to 40 minutes, then remove foil and bake for an additional 15 minutes, until cheese is golden brown. Remove from heat and let rest 10 minutes before serving.

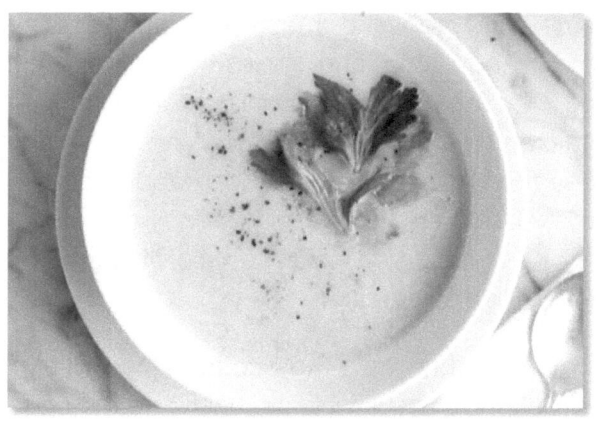

Tops and Bottoms Celery Soup

Tops and Bottoms Celery Soup

Ingredients:

- 2 tablespoons of olive oil or avocado oil

- one 1-pound celery root, peeled and cut into 1-inch cubes

- 2 celery stalks with leaves, cut into 1-inch pieces

- ½ chopped red onion

- 1/4 tablespoon chopped fresh rosemary leaves

- Pinch of iodized salt

- Pinch of Black Pepper

- 3 cups organic vegetable broth

- 1/2 lemon

- 3 tablespoons chopped flat-leaf parsley, for garnish

Instructions:

- In a massive Dutch oven or serious saucepan, heat the 3 tablespoons of olive oil over medium heat. Add the chopped celery root, celery, onion, rosemary, salt, and pepper, and cook for about 5 minutes, till the celery root and celery begin to melt and brown a small amount.

- Add the broth and lemon, and convey to a boil. Reduce the warmth, cowl, and simmer for thirty minutes. Stir often and check to see when the celery root is tender. Once it is, remove from heat.

- Transfer concerning 0.5 of the mixture to a high-speed blender and blend on the purée or soup setting until swish and creamy. Repeat with the remainder of the mixture and then reheat the entire batch in the Dutch oven for about 5 minutes. To serve, pour into serving bowls and garnish with parsley. Drizzle one tablespoon olive oil over every bowl, if desired.

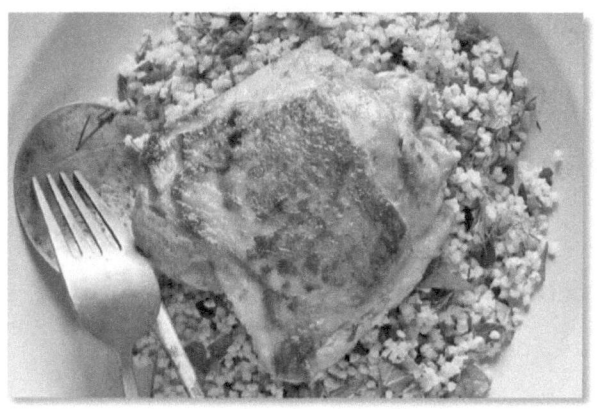

Moroccan Spiced Chicken with Millet Tabbouleh

Moroccan Spiced Chicken with Millet Tabbouleh

Ingredients:

- For the chicken
- 2 cups coconut yogurt, plain
- Juice of one lemon
- Zest of lemon
- Zest of one orange
- 1/2 teaspoon cinnamon
- 1/2 teaspoon cumin

- 1/2 teaspoon paprika

- 1/2 teaspoon black pepper

- 1/2 teaspoon Turmeric

- 1/2 teaspoon iodized sea salt

- 4 pasture-raised chicken thighs For the tabbouleh

- 2 cups cooked millet

- 1/2 cup minced parsley

- 1/2 cup minced meant

- 1/4 cup minced dill

- 1 teaspoon iodized sea salt

- 1 tablespoon extra-virgin all of oil

- Juice of one lemon

- 1/4 cup red wine vinegar

Instructions:

- Marinate the chicken: in a large Ziploc bag, mix the yogurt, lemon juice, lemon zest, orange zest, and spices. Add the chicken, and marinate for at least one hour. (If using temporary, use the same marinade, but for 30 minutes.)

- Preheat the oven to 375°F, prepare a broiler pan or a sheet tray with wire rack by spring with oil. Set aside.

- Make the tabbouleh: mix all ingredients in a large bowl, and stir well. Let the flavors meld for at least 20 minutes (which is perfect, since you need that time to cook the chicken).

- Remove chicken of bread and parentheses or tempeh) for marinade, pat dry with paper towels, and the range on the prepared baking sheet. If your chicken has skin, place it's going down.

- Bake the chicken for 20 to 25 minutes, then flip and bake for an additional 10 to 15 minutes, skin side up, and tell me it has reached

- 165°F and skin is crisp. Remove from heat, and left rest five minutes before serving.

- If using tempeh: bake for 12 to 15 minutes, flipping occasionally, until crispy. Remove from heat and serve immediately.

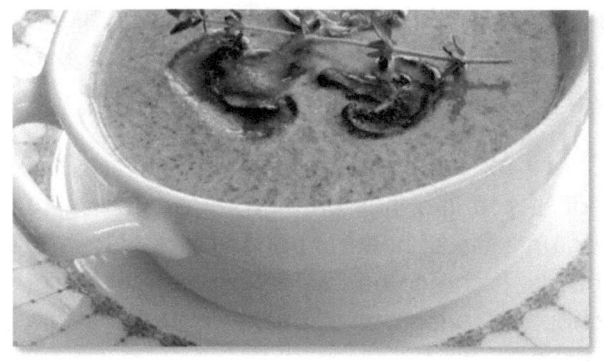

Amji's Special Vegetable Mushroom Soup

Amji's Special Vegetable Mushroom Soup

Ingredients:

- 1/2 cup of raw walnuts

- 3 teaspoons of dried minced onion

- Pinch of sea salt

- Pinch of Black Pepper

- 1/2 teaspoon dried thyme

Instructions:

• Chop 1/2 of cup of the mushrooms and set aside. Place the remaining 2 cups mushrooms, the water, walnuts, onions, salt, pepper, and thyme during a food processor with the S-blade or during a high-speed blender. Pulse for thirty seconds, and then mix for two minutes.

• Check for temperature-it should be heat however not hot. If you like, mix on high for another minute or longer, until it gets hotter. I pour or spoon the soup into two bowls. It should be thick and gravy- like. Top with the chopped mushrooms, drizzle with the truffle oil, if desired, and serve.

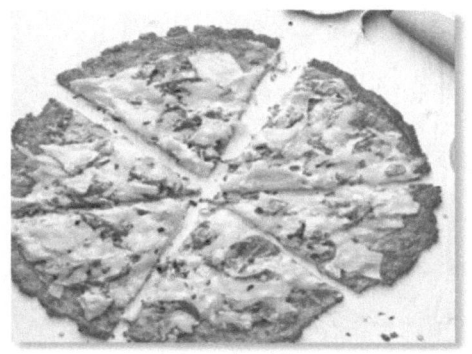

Hamzi's Pizza
(With thin crust of Cauliflowers)

Hamzi's Pizza

Ingredients:

For Crust

- Olive Oil

- 1 small head of chopped cauliflower

- omega-3 egg (Lightly bitten)

- 2 tablespoon of goat mozzarella

- Pinch of Iodized salt

- Pinch of Black Pepper

- Pinch dried oregano For Topping

- chopped vegetables (Your Choice)

- 1 cup of Romano cheese

- Pinch of Sea Salt

Instructions:

- Rinse the cauliflower. You may have approximately 3 cups. Transfer to a microwave-safe dish and microwave on high for 8 minutes, until cooked. Allow to chill, stirring sometimes. Place a rack in the center of the oven. Heat the oven to 450°f. Grease a ten-in. ovenproof frying pan with olive oil.

- Place the cooled riced cauliflower during a dishtowel, and twist and squeeze to get rid of all the moisture. Transfer to a mixing bowl. Add the egg, mozzarella, salt, pepper, and oregano. Combine well.

- Press the mixture evenly within the frying pan over medium heat on the stove high, crisp the cauliflower crust for some minutes. Transfer to the oven and bake for 15 minutes, until golden. Let cool for 5 minutes, and add the topping.

- Scatter the mozzarella evenly over the pizza base and spread the spinach. Add any additional vegetables. Sprinkle with the pecorino Romano cheese and add a pinch of salt. Bake for a further ten minutes, until the cheese has melted.

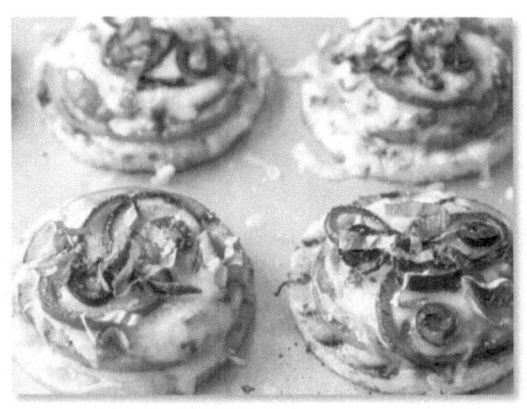

Mini Grilled Pizza (Pesto Special)

Mini Grilled Pizza

Ingredients:

For Basil pesto

- 1 cup of fresh basil leaves

- 2 tablespoon of olive oil

- 3 tablespoons of walnuts

- two 1-inch cubes parmigiano Reggiano For Mini "pizzas"

- 3 Pieces of chopped mushroom

- 2 slices of Italian prosciutto

- Pieces of Mozzarella

- Pinch of iodized Salt

- Pinch of Black Pepper

- 1/2-inch-thick slices

Instructions:

- Make the pesto. In a mini food processor, pulse the basil, olive oil, pine nuts, and cheese until well blended.

- Make the "pizzas." Set one burner of a gas grill to high or place a grill pan on the stove with burner set to medium-high heat with the exhaust fan on. Rub the cap aspect of the mushrooms with oil, place on the grill or grill pan, cap facet up, and grill for regarding 5 minutes, until the caps begin to brown slightly. Flip over and grill, gill side up, for an additional five minutes. Remove the mushrooms from the grill or burner. Leave the warmth on.

- Spoon 3 tablespoons of pesto onto the gill aspect of 1 mushroom, add one slice prosciutto, arranging it to suit neatly in the gill cup, and then top with half the mozzarella slices. Repeat with the other mushroom. If cooking on a grill, come back the mushrooms to the grill, shut the hood, and grill till the cheese begins to soften, about 5 minutes.

• If cooking indoors, return the grill pan to the stove top for about 5 minutes; alternatively, cover the grill pan with a glass casserole cover to "steam" for 5 minutes.

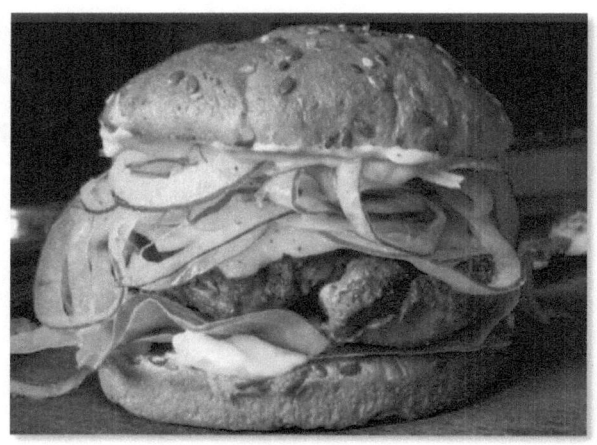

Vegetable and Meaty Burger (Rich Proteins)

Vegetable and Meaty Burger

Ingredients:

- A cup of walnuts

- 2 cups of chopped mushrooms

- 1 cup chopped red beet

- Pinch of garlic powder

- 1/2 cup of dried minced onions

- Pinch of paprika

- ¼ cup of dried parsley

- Pinch of Iodized Slat

- Pinch of black pepper

- 4 tablespoons of chopped fresh basil

- 6 teaspoons cassava or tapioca flour

- 1/3 cup of olive oil

- Some butter lettuce leaves

- 1 sliced hass avocado

Instructions:

- Put the walnuts, mushrooms, beet, garlic, 1/4 cup of the onion, paprika, dried parsley, 1/4. Teaspoon salt, and 1/4 teaspoon pepper in a food processor fitted with the s-blade. Pulse and blend until blended but still chunky.

- Transfer this mixture to a mixing bowl and stir in the basil, the remaining one/4 cup onion, and therefore grease your hands with olive oil and knead the mixture to completely combine ingredients. On a sheet of wax paper, kind into four patties, each about 4 inches in diameter and 1 in. thick. Use a low mug or lowball glass to form the patties, if you want.

• Heat a massive skillet over medium-high heat. Pour in 3 tablespoons of olive or avocado oil. Add the patties, cooking 4 to 5 minutes per aspect, till nicely browned. To serve, place every patty on a lettuce leaf, add a dollop of avocado mayo, if desired, add salt and pepper to style, top with slices of avocado, and cover with a second lettuce leaf.

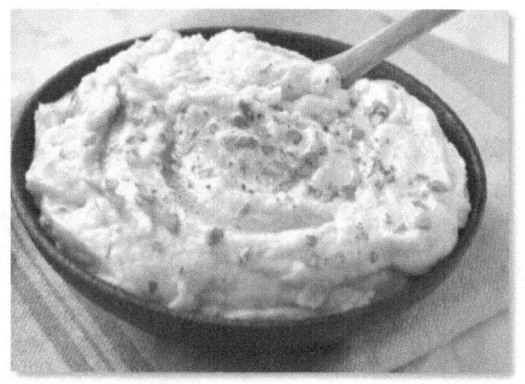

Meshed Roasted Cauliflowers

Meshed Roasted Cauliflowers

Ingredients:

- 1 large head of chopped cauliflower

- 4 tablespoons of olive oil

- Pinch of Iodized salt

- Pinch of black pepper

- ¼ cup of unsalted French or Italian butter

- 1 cup of Parmigiano Reggiano cheese

Instructions:

1 Heat the oven to 400°F. Place the cauliflower florets in a giant bowl, add the olive oil, and toss to coat well, seasoning generously with sea salt and black pepper. Lay a giant sheet of aluminum foil, shiny facet up, on the countertop. Fold in 0.5 and then reopen the foil.

•   Transfer the cauliflower to the center of one half of the foil. Fold over the other half and crimp the edges to seal the packet.

•   Place on a cookie sheet and position on the middle rack of the oven. Cook until very tender and slightly browned, about 1 hour. Remove from the over. Open the pouch carefully—do not let any juice flow out–and cool for about 10 minutes.

•   Transfer the cauliflower and its liquid to a food processor. Add the butter, if desired, and the Parmesan. Purée until smooth and thickened. Season with salt and pepper to taste. Serve immediately.

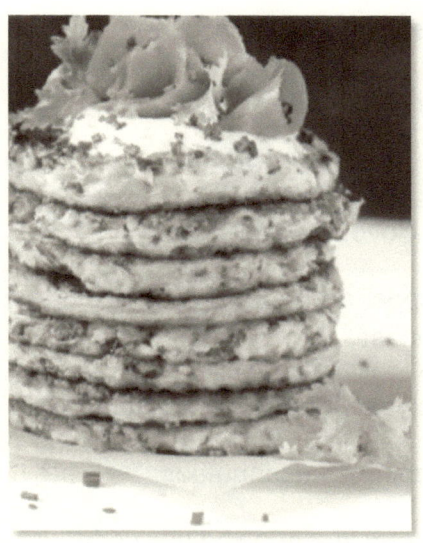

Fritters made with Cauliflowers with White Sauce

Fritters made with Cauliflowers with White Sauce

Ingredients:

- For the fritters

- 7 ounces (approximately 2 cups) cauliflower florettes, steamed until tender

- Two large omega-3 or pastured eggs or vegan eggs

- 2 tablespoons coconut yogurt

- Two green onions, finely chopped

- 1 tablespoon chopped parsley

- 1 tablespoon chopped mint

- 1 garlic clove, finely grated

- 2 tablespoons grated Parmesan cheese or nutritional yeast

- 5 to 6 tablespoons cassava flour

- 2 tablespoons coconut flour

- One quarter teaspoon baking soda

- 1 teaspoon iodized sea salt

- 1/8 teaspoon Pulver black pepper

- 3 to 4 tablespoons coconut oil for frying For the yogurt sauce

- 6 ounces coconut yogurt

- 2 tablespoons extra virgin olive oil

- 1 tablespoon tahini

- Juice of one-half lemon

- 1 teaspoon paprika

- Pinch of iodized sea salt

Instructions:

• In the work bowl of a food processor fitted with an S-blade, pulse the cauliflower, eggs, yogurt, green onion, parsley, mint, and garlic until finally crumbled and well mix.

• Transfer to a mixing bowl, then add the cheese or yeast and 2 tablespoons of cassava flour, coconut flour, baking soda, salt, and pepper, and mix again. Mixture should form a cohesive dough. If it's too runny, add more cassava flour, 1 teaspoon at a time

• Let the mixture rest for five minutes – the perfect opportunity to make the yogurt sauce.

• Mix together the yogurt, olive oil, tahini, lemon juice, paprika, and sea salt. Set aside until ready to serve.

• Heat the coconut oil in a medium skillet over medium heat.

• Spoon a tablespoon of batter in the pan. Flatten with the back of a spoon or spatula until approximately further shapes. Look For two minutes per side, flipping carefully. Do you know more than three or four fritters at a time to prevent the pan.

• Cook in batches until all the batter is used. Serve the fritters fresh out of the skillet with the yogurt sauce on the side.

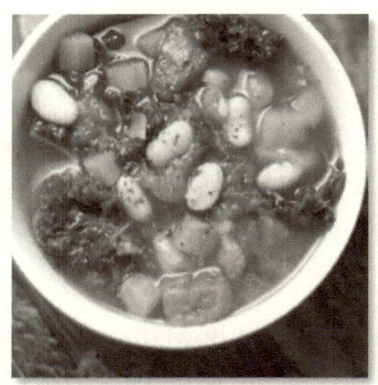

White Beans with Kale Soup
(Pressure Cooker)

White Beans with Kale Soup

Ingredients:

- 1 bunch of Tuscans

- 1 medium chopped red onion

- Pinch of Garlic Powder

- 1/3 cup of Olive oil

- 1-pound dried large lima beans, rinsed and picked through

- 4 cups vegetable stock or bone broth

- 3 of cups water

- 2 teaspoons Italian seasoning

- 1 small pastured bone-in turkey thigh, about 3/4 pound

- ¼ cup of grainy mustard

- Pinch of powdered sage

- Pinch of iodized salt

- Pinch of black pepper

- 1/2 cup of truffle oil

Instructions:

- Slice the leaves off the stems of the kale. Chop the stems and chop the leaves into larger items. Set aside. If your pressure cooker encompasses a saute feature, sauté the onions and the garlic in the oil for concerning 5 minutes.

- Alternatively, sauté them in a non-Teflon frying pan or wok over medium-heat. Transfer the garlic and onions to the pressure cooker. Add the vegetable stock and water. Add the beans, Italian seasoning, and turkey thigh.

- Cook at high pressure for fourteen minutes, then allow the pressure to come down naturally. Remove the turkey, and stir in the kale leaves, mustard, sage, and salt and pepper to taste. Shred the turkey and come back to the pot.

• Shake until well blended, and ladle into serving bowls. Drizzle each serving with a tablespoon of olive oil or truffle oil.

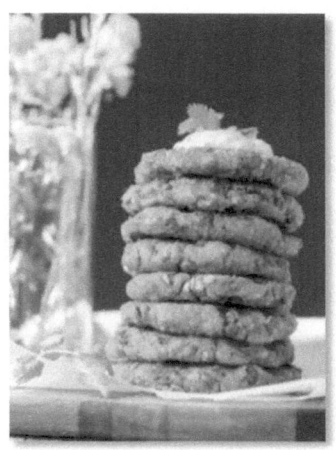

Lectin Free Sweet Potato Millet Cakes

Lectin Free Sweet Potato Millet Cakes

Ingredients:

- 4 tablespoons of millet

- 2 cups vegetable stock or water

- Pinch of Iodized Salt

- Pinch of Black Pepper

- 4 tablespoons of red onion

- 4 tablespoons of chopped carrots

- 4 tablespoons of chopped basil

- 4 tablespoons of chopped mushrooms

- 1 tablespoons of chopped garlic

- 1/2 teaspoon Italian seasoning

- 2 tablespoons extra-virgin olive oil or perilla oil

- 1 pastured or omega-3 egg, beaten

- 1 tablespoon coconut flour

Instructions:

- In a large dry saucepan, toast the millet over medium heat for about 5 minutes, stirring or shaking frequently, till golden brown and fragrant. Do not burn. Slowly add the vegetable stock and salt, being careful not to induce burned from the rising steam. Stir and produce to boil. Lower the heat to simmer, cover the pan, and cook for about 15 minutes, till all the water is absorbed.

- Remove from the heat and let stand covered for 10 minutes, then fluff with a fork. Meanwhile, place the onion, carrots, basil, mushrooms, garlic, and Italian seasoning in a food processor fitted with the S-blade and pulse into fine pieces.

- Place 1 tablespoon of the oil during a giant skillet over medium heat, add the vegetable mixture, and sauté for three to four, minutes, till tender. Transfer to a massive bowl. Wipe the skillet clean with a paper towel. Add the millet, beaten egg, and coconut flour to the mixing bowl. Stir to mix and thicken.

• With greased hands, form the mixture into 2- inch balls, and then press down with the palm of your hand to form into 12 patties. Add the remaining 1 tablespoon oil to the skillet. Add the patties and sauté over medium heat for 5 minutes per side. Drain on a paper-towel-covered plate before serving.

Chapter 5:

Desserts

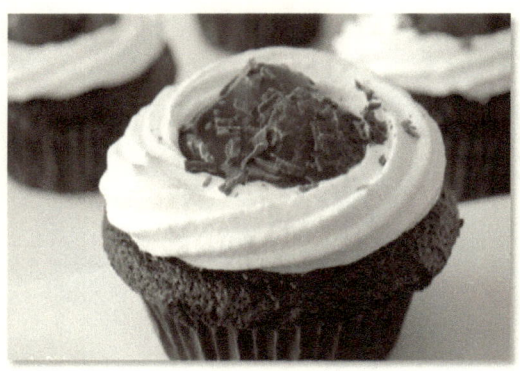

Cupcakes with Whipped Cream and Chocolate Frosting

Cupcakes with Whipped Cream and Chocolate Frosting

Our black forest cupcakes are light and fluffy, with the flavor of a dense chocolate cake. They're perfect for celebrating a special occasion…or just because!

Making your own whipped cream and cherry filling takes a bit more time, but it's totally worth it. You'll get a delicious, homemade flavor and no added sugars or gross preservatives.

Ingredients:

For Cake

- 3/4 cup cassava flour
- 1/3 cup natural cocoa powder

- 3/4 teaspoon baking soda
- 1/2 teaspoon salt
- 1/4 cup unsalted butter, plus more to grease pan
- 1/2 cup monk fruit/erythritol granulated sweetener
- pastured eggs
- 1/2 teaspoon pure vanilla extract
- 3/4 cup coconut milk + 1 tablespoon vinegar For Filling
- 1/4 cup Kirshwasser (Cherry brandy) or tart cherry juice
- 1/4 cup unsalted butter
- 1 cup monk fruit/erythritol granulated sweetener
- pinch of sea salt
- 1/8 cup espresso from a prepared liquid espresso
- 1-pound black cherries, pitted and halved For Topping
- 1 cup heavy whipping cream
- 1/4 teaspoon pure vanilla extract
- 1 tablespoon monk fruit/erythritol granulated sweetener
- 1/2 tablespoon Kirshwasser
- 1/4 cup bitter chocolate shavings

Instructions:

Do ahead: set aside 18-20 cherries for decoration, and soak the rest in 1/4 cup kirsch overnight.

For Cupcakes

• Preheat an oven to 350 degrees f.

• Grease an 18-cup cupcake pan with butter (do not use cupcake liners, as you'll be cutting them in half)

• Mix the vinegar and coconut milk together, and allow to sit for 10 minutes.

• Meanwhile, sift the dry cake ingredients together in a small bowl, and, in a separate large bowl, cream the butter and sweetener together. Add the eggs to the creamed mixture. Alternate adding dry mix and the vinegar-coconut milk to the large bowl, mixing well as you add.

• Pour batter evenly into cupcake cups. Start by adding one large spoonful at a time to each cup. Do not fill cups more than halfway. If there's extra batter, use an additional pan or work in batches. Bake for 15-20 minutes, until a toothpick inserted into the middle comes out clean. Cool and remove the cupcakes from the pan.

For Filling

• Beat the butter until light and creamy. Add the sweetener, salt, and espresso, and mix well. If the filling is too thick (not spreadable), add kirsch or cherry juice, 1 tablespoon at a time.

• Cut each cupcake in half. Pour 1 teaspoon of kirsch (that the cherries have soaked in) on the bottom half of each cupcake, then spread with a layer of filling, and a small handful of soaked cherries. Replace the top half of each cupcake on the layer of filling, to make a "cupcake sandwich."

For Topping

• Whip the cream, vanilla, sweetener, and kirsch in a cold bowl until it forms stiff peaks.

• Decorate the cupcakes using a pastry bag filled with the cream or a cake decorating tool. Alternatively, spoon whipped topping onto each cupcake and gently shape into a "mound." Place a decorative cherry and some chocolate shavings onto each cupcake.

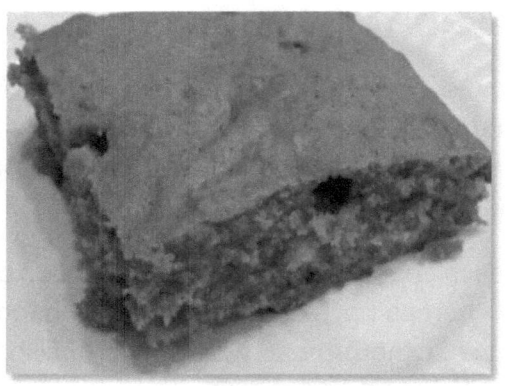

Potato Blondies with Cinnamon

Potato Blondies with Cinnamon

Ingredients:

- Olive oil or coconut oil spray
- 1/3 cup coconut oil, softened but not melted
- 1/3 cup yacon syrup or 4 tablespoons confectioners Swerve
- 1/2 cup sweet potato purée (from baked sweet potatoes)
- 1 cup coconut milk
- Two omega 3 or pasteured eggs or Vegan Eggs
- 2 cups blanched almond flour
- tablespoons coconut flour
- 1/2 teaspoon baking soda

- 1 teaspoon cinnamon

- 1/4 teaspoon cloves

- 1/2 teaspoon vanilla extract

- 1/2 teaspoon salt

Instructions:

- Preheat the oven to 350°. Grease the 8 x 8"glass baking dish with olive or coconut oil.

- Using a Mix or a mixing bowl, or in a stand mixer with a paddle attachment, cream together the coconut oil and yacon syrup (or Swerve).

- Mix in the sweet potato purée, coconut milk, and eggs.

- Add the flours, baking soda, spices, vanilla extract, and salt and mix well.

- Spread the batter evenly in the prepared baking dish.

- Bake for 45 minutes, or until a toothpick inserted into the center comes out clean, and the tops are golden brown.

- Let cool to room temperature before cutting. Stored at room temperature in an airtight container for 3 to 4 days.

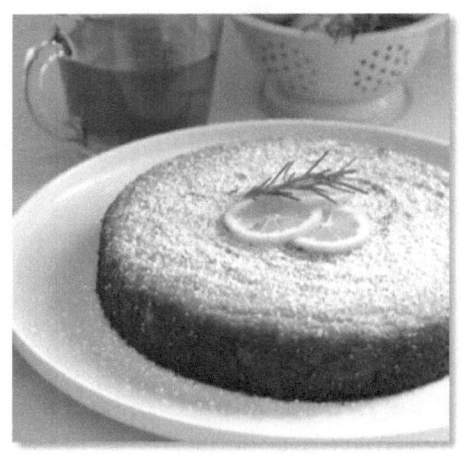

Olives Cake with Rosemary and Lemon

Olives Cake with Rosemary and Lemon

Ingredients:

- Olive oil spray

- 1 1/2 cups blanched almond flour

- Zest of one orange

- 2 Lemons

- tablespoons rosemary leaves, roughly chopped

- 1 cup xylitol

- teaspoons baking powder

- Zest of one lemon

- Juice of one lemon

- Do you thirds cup extra virgin olive oil

- For the syrup

- 1/2 cup water

- Juice of two lemons

- tablespoons xylitol

- Two sprigs of Rosemary

- To garnish

- Rosemary sprigs

- Goat's milk yogurt

- Grease an 8-inch cake tin with all of oil. (Ideally, use a springform pan).

Instructions:

- In a food processor fitted with an S-blade, pulse the almond flour, orange zest, and rosemary until they're as fine as possible.

- Transfer to a mixing bowl and stir in the xylitol,

baking powder, and lemon zest. Add the lemon juice, olive oil, and eggs and mix until mix.

• Pour the batter into prepared cake pan, then put into a cold oven. Turn the oven to 350°F, and bake for approximately 25 to 30 minutes, or until a skewer inserted into the center of the cake comes out clean.

• Leave in the tin for 5 to 10 minutes to cool.

• While the cake is cooling, make the syrup. Gently heat all of the ingredients in a small sauce pan over medium heat until the xylitol has dissolved.

• Bring to a gentle boil for five minutes, allowing the rosemary to infuse. Remove rosemary sprigs.

• Using a bamboo skewer or the end of a meat thermometer, pierce holes all over the cake. Pour the syrup over the cake while still warm.

• Once cool, serve garnished with rosemary sprigs and a dollop of goat's milk yogurt. Store leftovers in an airtight container at room temperature for 3 to 4 days.

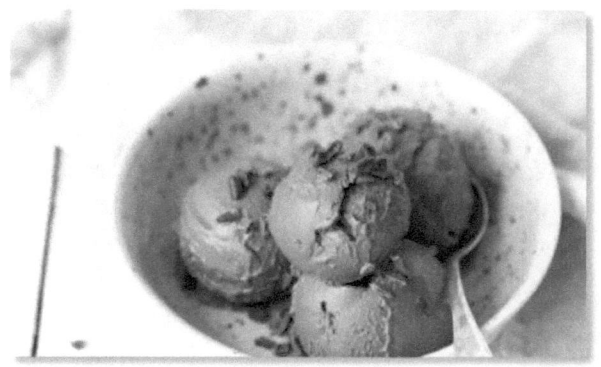

Chocolate Chip Avocado Ice-cream (Especially for Summer)

Chocolate Chip Avocado Ice-Cream

Ingredients:

- 15-ounce of coconut milk

- 2 tablespoons of sugar

- Pinch of Coffee Powder

- 2 tablespoons of coca powder

- 3 ounces (about one bar) 85% to 90% sugar- free dark chocolate, chopped

- ½ tablespoon of vanilla extract

- 2 Hass avocados, peeled and pits removed.

- ½ cup of chopped fresh mint, or 10 drops Sweet Leaf Mint Stevia drops, or to taste

- 1/2 cup 72% or more sugar-free extra-dark chocolate chips or 1/2 cup chopped 100% percent cocoa baking chocolate

Instructions:

- Put the coconut milk, sweetener, low powder, and cocoa powder in a medium saucepan. Mix over medium heat, until the sweetener has dissolved and therefore the mixture is mixed. Turn off the warmth. Add the chopped chocolate and stir till melted.

- Place the chocolate mixture in a very food processor fitted with the S-blade or a blender. Add the vanilla extract, avocados, and mint, and mix till smooth. Pour into a bowl, cover, and refrigerate for 2 hours, until cool.

- Stir in the chocolate chips until well dispersed. Spoon or pour into an ice cream maker (see Note) and churn until thick and set. It will be the consistency of sentimental-serve ice cream. Serve immediately. You'll be able to conjointly freeze to a firmer consistency and serve later: transfer to a metal or glass container and cover with wax paper secured with a rubber band.